Presented by Merck Sharp & Dohme

as a Service to Dermatologists

DIVISION OF MERCK & CO., INC., WEST POINT, PENNSYLVANIA 19486

Manual of
Dermatologic Syndromes

Thomas Butterworth, A.B., M.D., Med.Sc.M.

*Associate Professor of Dermatology,
University of Pennsylvania; Chief, Department of Dermatology, Pennhurst
State School; Emeritus Chief, Department of Dermatology, The Reading
Hospital; Consultant in Dermatology,
Pottstown Hospital, Berks County Tuberculosis Sanitorium.*

Second Edition

J. B. Lippincott Company
Philadelphia · Toronto

SP—B

1   3   5   7   8   6   4   2

To my wife Evelyn, a typically patient practitioner's help-mate, this manual is dedicated.

Preface

This enlarged revision of the Manual of Dermatologic Syndromes by Butterworth and Strean has been written primarily to fulfill the expanded needs and interests of the dermatologist. Since many of the syndromes described present osseous, ophthalmologic, pediatric, neurologic, endocrine, hematologic, metabolic and other manifestations, this ready reference volume may also prove valuable to specialists in many other fields of medicine. It is hoped that the brief presentation of the syndromes may afford diagnostic clues and help guide the clinician in the study of his patients.

Many new syndromes have been described by dermatologists in the past decade. While, in some instances, the entities have not consisted of "a set of symptoms which occur together," they have been accepted as syndromes by usage and the passage of time. Since it is my desire to inform and not reform, I have included such "pseudo-syndromes" in the text.

Dermatology is expanding upon an ever increasing base. The practitioner in this field has a keen interest in syndromes with dermatologic manifestations even though the chief complaint or disability lies in the field of another specialist. The increased use of consultations in hospital practice makes this knowledge of great practical importance. To meet this need I have "borrowed" many syndromes from other branches of medicine.

I wish to give recognition to the late Dr. Lyon P. Strean with whom I wrote the first edition of this manual. His untiring devotion and scientific curiosity were sorely missed in the present work. He helped build the foundation upon which this later edition has been enlarged.

I also wish to mention Miss Lois K. Mazur and Mrs. Helen Y. Clouse for their secretarial assistance in preparing the text and index respectively.

Thomas Butterworth

Introduction

A syndrome represents a complex of characteristic signs and symptoms that occur in close association. An unexplained factor is frequently involved, and the various manifestations appear to be linked together in some mysterious fashion. When seemingly unrelated pathologic conditions occur as a result of a known biochemical abnormality, the complex is recognized as a "disease." The term "syndrome" is a very convenient substitute for a description of a symptom-complex which would require a plethora of words to insure accuracy and clarity. This time-honored usage has proved acceptable even after a thorough understanding of the train of signs and symptoms should have established the complex as a disease.

Syndromes fall into one of two categories—eponymic or descriptive. In the former, the syndrome is identified by the name of one or more persons. The individuals so designated may have originally described the symptom complex or, by their studies, may have elucidated the clinical entity. Thus, several names may be associated with a particular syndrome. Descriptive syndromes are less common and, at times, more informative. For example, a functional disturbance, such as Familial Autonomic Dysfunction syndrome, is descriptive of a particular physiologic abnormality. The Nail-Patella-Elbow syndrome is indicative of anatomic changes. The Cat Scratch syndrome reveals the etiologic factor, while the Parotitis–herpangina–Coxsackie-virus syndrome refers to the location and the cause.

Some syndromes bear one or several eponymic designations and, in addition, one or more descriptive terms. This unfortunate situation results in confusion for the student and practitioner. Minor variations of established syndromes have been recorded as new syndromes, which results in more confusion.

The author has attempted to bring some order out of this chaos. More than 335 syndromes were selected for inclusion in this volume. Many of the better known of the multitudinous synonyms for these syndromes have been listed. No doubt there will be errors of omission and of commission; however, the main objective from the very outset has been satisfied—that is, to compile in one small pocket manual the cardinal features of selected dermatologic syndromes.

Syndromes

Acatalasemia
See Takahara's syndrome

Achard-Thiers Syndrome
syn: Diabetic–bearded women syndrome
1–Diabetes mellitus
2–Facial hirsutism and other signs of masculinization in women
3–Obesity
4–Hypertension

Achenbach's Syndrome
1–Sudden hematoma of palm
2–Piercing pain
3–Circumscribed edema

Acrodermatitis Enteropathica Syndrome
syn: Brandt's syndrome
Danbolt-Closs syndrome
1–Acral and periorificial dermatitis
2–Gastrointestinal disturbances
3–Alopecia

Acute Defibrination Syndrome
1–Ecchymoses into the skin
2–Areas of gangrene
3–Absence of plasma fibrinogen

Acute Febrile Neutrophilic Dermatosis
See Sweet's syndrome

Addisonian Syndrome
syn: Adrenocortical insufficiency syndrome
1–Mental, muscular, and cardiovascular asthenia
2–Diarrhea and digestive disturbances
3–Bronzelike pigmentation of the skin and mucous membranes
4–Progressive anemia

Adie's Syndrome
1–Tonicity of the pupils
2–Absence of tendon reflexes

Adrenal Virilism Syndrome
See Adrenogenital syndrome

Adrenocortical Insufficiency Syndrome
See Addisonian syndrome

Adrenogenital Syndrome
syn: Adrenal virilism syndrome
1–Increased production of androgens
2–Masculinization in the female
3–Sexual precocity in the male

Aigner's Syndrome
1–Punctate palmoplantar keratoses
2–Osteopoikilosis

Albright-McCune-Sternberg Syndrome
See Albright's syndrome

Albright's Syndrome
syn: Albright-McCune-Sternberg syndrome
      Wright's syndrome
1–Melanotic pigmentation of the skin
2–Osteitis fibrosa cystica
3–Precocious puberty in the female

Aldrich's Syndrome
See Wiskott-Aldrich syndrome

Alezzandrini's Syndrome
1–Unilateral degenerative retinitis
2–Ipsilateral vitiligo on face
3–Ipsilateral poliosis
4–Deafness may be present

Alibert-Bazin Syndrome
1–Granuloma fungoides

Allergic Dermal–Respiratory Syndrome
1–Urticaria or eczema
2–Asthma, hay fever, or perennial rhinitis

Allergic Granulomatosis Syndrome
See Churg-Strauss syndrome

Angioendotheliomatosis Proliferans Systemisata Syndrome
1–Chills and fever
2–Nodules of various sizes on the trunk and extremities
3–Diffuse malignant proliferation of vascular endothelium

Angiokeratoma Corporis Diffusum
See Fabry-Anderson syndrome

Angiomatosis Retinae et Cerebelli Syndrome
See von Hippel-Lindau syndrome

Anterior Tibial Syndrome
1–Embolism or thrombosis of the anterior tibial artery
2–Sudden severe pain in the anterior tibial compartment
3–Swelling, tenderness, reddish-blue discoloration and ischemic necrosis

Arachnodactyly Syndrome
See Marfan's syndrome

Arndt-Gottron Syndrome
syn: Scleromyxedema
1–Lichen myxedematosus
2–Diffuse thickening of the skin

Ascher's Syndrome
1–Edema of the upper eyelids
2–Blepharochalasis
3–Hyperplastic labial glands and tissues
4–Acquired "double" lip

Ataxia-Telangiectasia Syndrome
syn: Cephalo-oculocutaneous-telangiectasia syndrome
Louis Bar syndrome
1–Progressive cerebellar ataxia
2–Oculocutaneous telangiectasia
3–Peculiar eye movements
4–Frequent sinopulmonary infections

4

Auriculotemporal Syndrome

syn: Frey's syndrome

1–Pain, vasodilatation, and hyperhidrosis of the cheek while eating

Autoerythrocyte Sensitization Syndrome

syn: Gardner-Diamond syndrome
Painful bruising syndrome
Psychogenic purpura

1–Painful ecchymoses
2–Neurological and psychiatric symptoms
3–Abdominal pain
4–Menometrorrhagia
5–Gastrointestinal bleeding

Babinski's Syndrome

1–Late syphilis
2–Cardiac and arterial lesions

Bamatter's Syndrome

1–Progeria
2–Nanism
3–Microcornea
4–Corneal opacity
5–Enlarged joints
6–Generalized osseous dysplasia
7–Flabby skin
8–Tooth discoloration

Barré-Masson Syndrome

1–Glomangioma

Bart-Pumphrey Syndrome

1–Knuckle pads
2–Total leukonychia
3–Deafness

Bean-Maffucci Syndrome
See Maffucci's syndrome

Bean's Syndrome
See Blue rubber-bleb nevus syndrome

Behçet's Syndrome
syn: Cutaneomucouveal syndrome
1–Recurrent ulceration of the genitals
2–Intermittent aphthous lesions of the mouth
3–Uveitis or iridocyclitis followed by hypopyon

Berardinelli's Syndrome
See Lipoatrophic diabetes syndrome

Berlin's Syndrome
1–Facies resembles that of anhidrotic ectodermal dysplasia
2–Mental and physical retardation
3–Delayed dentition but teeth are not conical
4–Generalized mottled pigmentation of the fine dry skin
5–Thickening of the palms and soles
6–Pubic and axillary hair are sparse and vellus is sparse or absent
7–Sweating may be reduced

Bernard-Horner Syndrome
See Horner's syndrome

Bjornstad's Syndrome
1–Pili torti
2–Deafness of the cochlear type

Blegvad-Haxthausen Syndrome
1–Blue sclerae
2–Brittle bones
3–Macular atrophy
4–Cataracts
5–Deafness

Bloch-Siemens Syndrome
See Bloch-Sulzberger syndrome

Bloch-Sulzberger Syndrome
syn: Bloch-Siemens syndrome
    Incontinentia pigmenti syndrome
1–Irregular pigmentation often preceded by bullous or verrucous phases
2–Neurological, mental, bony, ocular, and dental defects

Bloom's Syndrome
1–Primordial dwarfs
2–Telangiectatic erythematous areas resembling lupus erythematosus on face
3–Crusted bullous lesions on lips
4–Sun sensitivity
5–Café-au-lait spots

Blue Rubber-Bleb Nevus Syndrome
syn: Bean's syndrome
1–Bluish bladderlike hemangiomas of the skin
2–Spontaneous nocturnal pain
3–Supralesional sweating
4–Bleeding from intestinal hemangiomas

Bogorad's Syndrome
See Crocodile tear syndrome

Bonnet-Dechaume-Blanc Syndrome
1–Telangiectatic facial nevus
2–Retinal and intracranial angiomatosis predominantly around the thalamus and mesencephalon

Bonnevie-Ullrich Syndrome
See Turner's syndrome

Böök's Syndrome
See PHC syndrome

Bourneville's Syndrome
See Pringle's syndrome

Brachmann-de Lange Syndrome
syn: Cornelia de Lange syndrome
1–Primordial growth failure
2–Various skeletal abnormalities
3–Mental retardation
4–Characteristic cry
5–Hirsutism
6–Cutis marmorata and facial "cyanosis"

Brandt's Syndrome
See Acrodermatitis enteropathica syndrome

Broad Thumb and Great Toe Syndrome
See Rubenstein-Taybi syndrome

Bronze Diabetes Syndrome
See Hanot-Chauffard syndrome

Brugsch's Syndrome
Probably same as Touraine-Solente-Golé syndrome

Brünauer Syndrome
1–Palmoplantar keratosis
2–Mental retardation
3–Defective enamel formation
4–Hyperhidrosis

Brunsting's Syndrome
1–Chronic herpetiform plaques about the head and neck
2–Atrophic scarring of the affected sites
3–Severe burning and itching
4–Mostly middle-aged or older men

Brushfield-Wyatt Syndrome
1–Extensive port-wine staining of the skin
2–Hemiplegia
3–Mental retardation
4–Various stigmata of degeneration

Bureau-Barriere Syndrome
1–Thermoanesthesia
2–Ulceration of the foot
3–Osteolysis with progressive deformity, notably shortening
4–Hyperhidrosis
5–Tactile anesthesia and analgesia may occur

Bureau-Barriere-Thomas Syndrome

syn: Thomas-Bureau syndrome
1–Orthopedic abnormalities
2–Clubbing of fingers and toes
3–Diffuse palmoplantar keratosis
4–Peculiarly tall individuals

Bürger-Grütz Syndrome

syn: Idiopathic familial hyperlipemia syndrome
1–Xanthomas of skin and mucous membranes
2–Hepatosplenomegaly
3–Lipemia retinalis
4–Recurrent attacks of abdominal pain

Burning-Feet Syndrome

1–Burning pain in the feet
2–Vitamin deficiency

Buschke-Ollendorff Syndrome

1–Multiple cutaneous fibromas
2–Osteopoikilosis

Caffey's Syndrome

1–Hypervitaminosis-A

Candidiasis-Thymoma Syndrome

1–Generalized cutaneous candidiasis
2–Thymoma

Carcinoid Syndrome
syn: Thorson-Biörck syndrome
1–Peripheral vasomotor phenomena, notably peculiar flushing and episodic cyanosis
2–Asthma
3–Refractory diarrhea
4–Cardiac symptoms
5–Pellagrinoid dermatitis
6–Sclerodermalike changes of the lower extremities

Cardiocutaneous Syndrome
See Multiple lentigines syndrome

Carini's Syndrome
1–Collodion baby

Cartilage-Hair Hypoplasia
See McKusick's syndrome

Cassirer's Syndrome
1–Acrocyanosis

Cat Scratch Syndrome
1–Red, tender papule at the site of a cat scratch
2–Regional lymphadenopathy
3–Irregular fever
4–Systemic manifestations

Cephalo-oculocutaneous Telangiectasia Syndrome
See Ataxia-telangiectasia syndrome

Cervical Rib Syndrome
See Scalenus anticus syndrome

Cervical Sympathetic Paralysis Syndrome
See Horner's syndrome

Cervico-oculo-acoustic Syndrome
syn: Wildervanck's syndrome
1–Stiff short neck
2–Low implantation of hair
3–Deafness
4–Abducens paralysis
5–Retraction of the bulb

Chand Syndrome
1–Curly hair
2–Ankyloblepharon
3–Nail dysplasia

Chediak-Higashi Syndrome
1–Anomalous leukocytic inclusions
2–Photophobia, pale ocular fundi, and decreased lacrimation
3–Hyperhidrosis
4–Pigmentary disturbances: oculocutaneous albinism and excessive pigmentation of areas exposed to sunlight
5–Hepatosplenomegaly and lymphadenopathy

Chlorpromazine Syndrome
syn: Purple people syndrome
Skin-eye syndrome
1–Light brown, slate gray, or violaceous discoloration of the exposed parts
2–Deposition of fine particulate matter in the cornea and lens
3–Star shaped opacities in the anterior portion of the lens

Chondrodystrophia Congenita Punctata Syndrome
See Conradi's syndrome

Chondroectodermal Dysplasia Syndrome
See Ellis–van Creveld syndrome

Christ-Siemens Syndrome
syn: Christ-Siemens-Touraine syndrome
Weech's syndrome
1–Anhidrotic ectodermal dysplasia

Christ-Siemens-Touraine Syndrome
See Christ-Siemens syndrome

Chronic Familial Neutropenia Syndrome
1–Constant depression of neutrophil count
2–Marked periodontal lesions

Churg-Strauss Syndrome
syn: Allergic granulomatosis syndrome
1–Debilitation
2–Attacks of fever
3–Eosinophilia
4–Asthma, ulcerative colitis, or organic disease of the heart and spleen
5–Erythematous papules or nodules on the extensor surfaces of the extremities and scalp

Clouston's Syndrome
syn: Hidrotic ectodermal dysplasia syndrome
1–Generalized hypotrichosis
2–Dystrophy of the nails
3–Hyperkeratosis of the palms and soles
4–Pigmentation

Cobb's Syndrome
 1–Venous hemangioma of spinal cord
 2–Port-wine stain of corresponding spinal segment of skin

Cockayne's Syndrome
 1–Lupus erythematosuslike dermatitis
 2–Atrophy of subcutaneous fat
 3–Defective mental and physical development
 4–Various ocular manifestations
 5–Progressive loss of hearing

Colcott Fox Syndrome
 1–Periporitis
 2–Abscess formation

Cole-Rauschkolb-Toomey Syndrome
 See Dyskeratosis congenita syndrome

Comedo-Cataract Syndrome
 1–Unilateral comedo nevus
 2–Ipsilateral uniocular congenital cataract

Congenital Iliac Horns Syndrome
 See Nail-patella-elbow syndrome

Conradi's Syndrome
 syn: Chondrodystrophia congenita punctata syndrome
 1–Stippled foci of calcification within hyaline cartilage
 2–Dwarfing
 3–Stiff contracted joints
 4–Congenital cataracts
 5–Ichthyosis
 6–Few and rudimentary hairs, eyebrows, and eyelashes

Cooked Hand Syndrome
1–Redness, swelling and stiffness following excessive use of heat after hand injuries

Cornelia de Lange Syndrome
See Brachmann-de Lange syndrome

Crigler-Najjar Syndrome
syn: Familial nonhemolytic jaundice with kernicterus syndrome
    Kernicterus syndrome
1–Marked retention icterus
2–Severe neurological disease

Crocodile Tear Syndrome
syn: Bogorad's syndrome
1–Paroxysmal lacrimation during eating as a sequel of facial palsy

Cronkhite-Canada Syndrome
1–Gastrointestinal polyposis
2–Generalized alopecia
3–Diffuse and spotty pigmentation
4–Atrophy of the nails
5–Diarrhea

CRST Syndrome
syn: Profichet's syndrome
    Scleroderma-calcinosis syndrome
    Thibierge-Weissenbach syndrome
1–Subcutaneous calcinosis
2–Raynaud's phenomenon
3–Sclerodactyly
4–Multiple telangiectasia

Cruveilhier-Baumgarten Syndrome
1–Guttate areas of hyperpigmentation on the abdomen and lower extremities
2–Keratotic papules on the palms and soles
3–Hepatosplenomegaly
4–Ascites
5–Cirrhosis of liver

Cryptophthalmia Syndrome
1–Extension of the skin of the forehead to completely cover one or both eyes
2–Total or partial soft tissue syndactyly of fingers or toes or both
3–Coloboma of the ala nasi
4–Abnormal hairline
5–Various urological abnormalities

Curtius' Syndrome
syn: Steiner's syndrome
1–Hemihypertrophy of the face with or without enlargement of half of the body
2–Thickening and pigmentation of skin of involved side with increased function of the sebaceous and sweat glands
3–Nevi
4–Telangiectasia

Cushing's Syndrome
1–Hirsutism
2–Acne
3–Abdominal striae
4–Moon face
5–"Buffalo hump" obesity
6–Mild insulin-resistant diabetes
7–Arterial hypertension

Cutaneo-auriculo-renal Syndrome
1–Ichthyosis
2–Neurosensory hearing loss
3–Renal disease
4–Prolinuria

Cutaneointestinal Syndrome
See Degos' syndrome

Cutaneomucouveal Syndrome
See Behçet's syndrome

Cutis Hyperelastica Syndrome
See Ehlers-Danlos syndrome

Danbolt-Closs Syndrome
See Acrodermatitis enteropathica syndrome

Degos' Syndrome
syn: Cutaneointestinal syndrome
    Malignant atrophic papulosis
1–Crops of crusted umbilicated papules
2–Depressed atrophic scars
3–Acute abdominal symptoms
4–Fatal fulminating peritonitis

Dennie-Marfan Syndrome
1–Congenital syphilis
2–Spastic paralysis
3–Mental retardation

Dercum's Syndrome
1–Multiple, painful, symmetrical lipomas
2–Obesity
3–Neuritis
4–Mental depression and deterioration

DeSanctis-Cacchione Syndrome
1–Xeroderma pigmentosum
2–Mental deficiency
3–Stunted growth
4–Occasional gonadal immaturity
5–Dyslalia

Diabetic–Bearded Women Syndrome
See Archard-Thiers syndrome

Donohue's Syndrome
syn: Leprechaunism
1–Hirsutism, especially facial
2–Retarded somatic and mental development with large genitalia

Down's Syndrome
syn: Mongolism
     Trisomy 21 anomaly
1–Mental retardation
2–Brachycephaly
3–Acromicria
4–Characteristic changes in skin, mucosae, hair, and eyes

Dresbach's Syndrome
See Sickle-cell disease

Dubin-Johnson Syndrome

  1–Chronic idiopathic icterus
  2–Greenish-black discoloration of liver

Dubowitz's Syndrome

  1–Small stature
  2–Peculiar facies
  3–Eczematoid skin eruption
  4–Thick skin
  5–Sparse hair

Dury–van Bogaert Syndrome

  1–Spastic diplegia
  2–Epilepsy
  3–Mental retardation
  4–Cutis marmorata
  5–Acrocyanosis
  6–Dystrophy of the nails
  7–Sometimes hypertrichosis

Dyschondroplasia with Hemangiomas Syndrome

  See Maffucci's syndrome

Dyskeratosis Congenita Syndrome

  syn: Cole-Rauschkolb-Toomey syndrome
      Zinsser-Cole-Engman syndrome
      Zinsser-Fanconi syndrome
  1–Atrophy and pigmentation of skin
  2–Dystrophy of nails and teeth
  3–Oral leukoplakia and sometimes bullae
  4–Various ocular manifestations

Dysplasia Oculodentodigitalis Syndrome

syn: Meyer-Schwickerath-Grüterich-Weyers syndrome
1–Microphthalmos, bilateral medial epicanthus, high myopia, glaucoma
2–Enamel defect, microdontia, missing teeth
3–Camptodactylia of the fifth fingers, variable syndactyly, missing middle phalanges of the toes
4–Hypotrichosis of the scalp, eyebrows, eyelashes; cutaneous atrophy
5–Small alae nasi with anteverted nostrils

Ectodermosis Erosiva Pluriorificialis Syndrome

See Stevens-Johnson syndrome

Ehlers-Danlos Syndrome

syn: Cutis hyperelastica syndrome
1–Hyperextensibility of joints
2–Hyperelasticity and friability of the skin
3–Fragility of blood vessels
4–Papyraceous scars
5–Pseudotumors
6–Spherules

Ehrlich-Fanconi Syndrome

See Fanconi's syndrome

Elastoidosis Syndrome

1–Numerous small cutaneous cysts, nodules, and comedones
2–Abnormal folds and wrinkles on face, neck, and ears

Ellis-van Creveld Syndrome

syn: Chondroectodermal dysplasia syndrome

1–Ectodermal dysplasia affecting the nails, hair, and teeth
2–Chondrodysplasia
3–Polydactyly
4–Congenital cardiac defect

Encephalotrigeminal Angiomatosis Syndrome

See Sturge-Weber syndrome

Epidemic Exfoliative Dermatitis Syndrome

See Savill's syndrome

Epidermal Nevus Syndrome

1–Epidermal nevus
2–Congenital skeletal disorders
3–Central nervous system disease

Epiloia

See Pringle's syndrome

Erb's Syndrome

1–Syphilitic spastic spinal paralysis

Erythema Multiforme Exudativum Major Syndrome

See Stevens-Johnson syndrome

Erythema Nodosum-Hilar Adenopathy Syndrome

1–Erythema nodosum
2–Bilateral hilar lymphadenopathy

Erythrokeratodermia Variabilis
See Mendes Da Costa's syndrome (1)

Fabry-Anderson Syndrome
syn: Angiokeratoma corporis diffusum
Ruiter-Pompen syndrome
Ruiter-Pompen-Wyers syndrome
1–Angiokeratoma of skin
2–Pain in the extremities
3–Disturbance in sweat secretion
4–Elevated blood pressure
5–Heart enlargement
6–Albuminuria

Familial Autonomic Dysfunction Syndrome
See Riley-Day syndrome

Familial Dysautonomia Syndrome
See Riley-Day syndrome

Familial Hypolipidemia
See Hooft's syndrome

Familial Idiopathic Dysproteinemia Syndrome
1–Familial edema of legs
2–Leg ulcers in males
3–Functional vascular changes in females

Familial Mediterranean Fever Syndrome
See Familial recurring polyserositis syndrome

Familial Mutilating Ulcerous Acropathy Syndrome
See Thévenard's syndrome

Familial Nonhemolytic Jaundice with Kernicterus Syndrome
See Crigler–Najjar syndrome

Familial Recurring Polyserositis Syndrome
syn: Familial Mediterranean fever syndrome
1–Short recurrent bouts of fever
2–Pain in abdomen and/or chest and/or joints
3–Erysipelaslike erythema

Familial Ulceration of the Extremities Syndrome
See Thévenard's syndrome

Fanconi's Syndrome
syn: Ehrlich-Fanconi syndrome
1–Severe progressive refractory hypoplastic anemia
2–Generalized brown pigmentation of the skin
3–Various congenital defects

Favre-Racouchot Syndrome
1–Senile atrophy of the skin
2–Epidermal cysts
3–Comedones

Feer's Syndrome
syn: Swift's syndrome
1–Acrodynia

Fegeler's Syndrome
syn: Post-traumatic nevus flammeus
1–Port-wine stain of the face
2–Ipsilateral weakness and hyperesthesia of the arm and leg
3–History of head injury

Feldman's Syndrome
See Graham Little syndrome

Felty's Syndrome
1–Chronic deforming arthritis
2–Splenomegaly and lymphadenopathy
3–Leukopenia
4–Nodules and pigmentation of skin
5–Leg ulcers

Fiessinger-Rendu Syndrome
See Stevens-Johnson syndrome

Fischer-Volavsek Syndrome
1–Palmoplantar keratosis
2–Onychogryposis or onycholysis
3–Sparse hair of scalp, brows, and lashes
4–Clubbing of fingers and toes
5–Hyperhidrosis of the hands and feet
6–Syringomyelia

Focal Dermal Hypoplasia Syndrome
syn: Goltz's syndrome
1–Linear areas of pigmentation and thinning of the skin with herniation of adipose tissue
2–Papillomatosis of the mucous membranes and skin
3–Dystrophy of the nails
4–Defects of the eyes, bones, teeth, heart, and central nervous system

Fong's Syndrome
See Nail-patella-elbow syndrome

Franceschetti-Jadassohn Syndrome
See Naegeli's syndrome

François Syndrome
See Hallermann-Streiff syndrome

Frey's Syndrome
See Auriculotemporal syndrome

Gammel's Syndrome
1–Erythema gyratum repens
2–May be associated with malignant disease

Gardner-Diamond Syndrome
See Autoerythrocytic sensitization syndrome

Gardner's Syndrome
1–Multiple polyposis of colon
2–Bony exostoses
3–Soft tissue tumors

Gargoylism
See Hurler's syndrome

Gaucher's Syndrome
1–Hepatosplenomegaly
2–Brown pigmentation of skin
3–Mucocutaneous hemorrhage
4–Cuneiform thickenings of ocular conjunctiva

Gianotti-Crosti Syndrome
syn: Infantile acrodermatitis papulosa syndrome
1–Erythematopapular lesions on face, neck, and extremities of children
2–Respiratory or gastrointestinal symptoms
3–Lymphadenopathy
4–Fever and malaise

Gideon-Gurish Syndrome
1–Loss of hair of scalp and eyebrows
2–Pear shaped nose
3–Deviation of fingers and toes

Glomangiomatous-osseous Malformation Syndrome
1–Multiple glomus tumors
2–Hypoplasia and osteoporosis of the bones of the affected forearm

Godfried-Prick-Carol-Prakken Syndrome
1–von Recklinghausen's disease
2–Atrophoderma vermiculatum
3–Mongoloid facies
4–Mental retardation
5–Heart abnormalities

Goldscheider's Syndrome
1–Dystrophic epidermolysis bullosa

Goltz's Syndrome
See Focal dermal hypoplasia syndrome

Gonococcal Dermatitis Syndrome
1–Intermittent fever
2–Arthralgia
3–Hemorrhagic vesicopustular eruption

Gopalan's Syndrome
1–Malnutrition
2–Burning and prickling sensation in extremities
3–Hyperhidrosis

Gorlin-Chaudhry-Moss Syndrome
1–Craniofacial dysostosis
2–Patent ductus arteriosus
3–Hypertrichosis
4–Hypoplasia of the labia majora
5–Dental and ocular abnormalities

Gorlin-Psaume Syndrome
See Oral-facial-digital syndrome

Gorlin's Syndrome
See Nevoid basal cell carcinoma syndrome

Gougerot-Blum Syndrome
1–Pigmented purpuric lichenoid dermatitis

Gougerot-Carteaud Syndrome
1–Confluent and reticulate papillomatosis

Gougerot-Mulock-Houwer Syndrome
See Sjögren's syndrome

Gougerot-Sjögren Syndrome
See Sjögren's syndrome

Gougerot Trisymptomatic Syndrome
1–Papuloerythematous rash resembling erythema multiforme
2–Purpuric macules
3–Discrete dermal or hypodermal nodules

Graham Little Syndrome
syn: Feldman's syndrome
     Lassueur–Graham Little syndrome
1–Lichen planus
2–Acuminate follicular papules
3–Cicatricial alopecia

Granuloma Fungoides
See Alibert-Bazin syndrome

Greither's Syndrome
1–Progressive diffuse thickening of palms and soles beginning in infancy
2–Warty keratoses on dorsa of the hands, feet, arms, and legs
3–Poikiloderma of face, hands, feet, forearms, and legs

Grönblad-Strandberg Syndrome
1–Pseudoxanthoma elasticum
2–Angioid streaks of retina

Gunther's Syndrome
1–Congenital erythropoietic porphyria

H-Disease
See Hartnup syndrome

H. Fischer's Syndrome
1–Hypotrichosis
2–Palmar and plantar hyperkeratosis with hyperhidrosis
3–Onychogryposis

Haber's Syndrome
1–Persistent familial rosacealike eruption of the face
2–Intraepidermal epitheliomata of the covered parts

Half and Half Nail Syndrome
1–White proximally; red, pink, or brown distally
2–Kidney disease, often azotemia

Hallermann-Streiff Syndrome
syn: François syndrome
1–Malformation of the skull
2–Proportionate nanism
3–Hypotrichosis
4–Atrophy of skin
5–Congenital cataracts

Hand-Foot Syndrome
1–Painful symmetrical swelling of hands or feet or both
2–Sickle-cell disease
3–Periosteal elevation or lytic areas or both, in the metacarpals, metatarsals, and phalanges

Hand-Schüller-Christian Syndrome
1–Defects in the membranous bones
2–Exophthalmos
3–Diabetes insipidus
4–Cutaneous xanthoma
5–Stomatitis and gingivitis

Hanhart's Syndrome
1–Diffuse palmoplantar keratosis which eventually appears elsewhere
2–Subcutaneous lipomas
3–Dendritic keratitis
4–Mental retardation

Hanot-Chauffard Syndrome
syn: Bronze diabetes syndrome
1–Diabetes mellitus
2–Hypertrophic cirrhosis of liver
3–Dark brown pigmentation of skin

Hart Syndrome
See Hartnup syndrome

Hartnup Syndrome
syn: Hart syndrome
"H" disease
1–Pellagralike skin rash
2–Intermittent cerebellar ataxia
3–Psychiatric manifestations
4–Constant aminoaciduria
5–Sensitive to sunlight

Haxthausen's Syndrome
1–Keratoderma climactericum
2–Obesity
3–Arterial hypertension

Heerfordt's Syndrome
1–Sarcoidosis
2–Enlargement of the parotid and lacrimal glands
3–Uveitis
4–Fever

Helweg-Larssen Syndrome
1–Congenital anhidrosis or severe hypohidrosis
2–Neurolabyrinthitis developing in the 4th or 5th
decade

Hemangioma-Thrombocytopenia Syndrome
syn: Kasabach-Merritt syndrome
1–Giant vascular tumor
2–Thrombocytopenia purpura

Hepato-cutaneous Syndrome
1–Juvenile cirrhosis
2–Allergic capillaritis of the skin
3–Proctocolitis
4–Arthritis

Hepatolenticular Degeneration Syndrome
See Wilson's syndrome

Hereditary Anhidrotic Ectodermal Dysplasia Syndrome
See Siemens' syndrome (1)

Hereditary Benign Intraepithelial Dyskeratosis Syndrome

syn: Witkop-Sallmann syndrome
1–Soft, white asymptomatic thickenings of oral mucosa
2–Bulbar conjunctivitis

Hereditary Hemorrhagic Telangiectasia Syndrome

See Rendu-Osler-Weber syndrome

Hereditary Onycho-osteodysplasia Syndrome

See Nail-patella-elbow syndrome

Hermansky-Pudlak Syndrome

1–Incomplete albinism
2–Pseudohemophilia

Herpes Zoster-Hemiplegia Syndrome

1–Herpes zoster ophthalmicus
2–Contralateral hemiplegia developing about four
   weeks later

Herrick's Syndrome

See Sickle-cell disease

Hidrotic Ectodermal Dysplasia Syndrome

See Clouston's syndrome

Hines-Bannick Syndrome

1–Intermittent attacks of low temperature and
   disabling sweating

Hooft's Syndrome
syn: Familial hypolipidemia
1–Retardation of growth
2–Erythematosquamous rash on face and extremities
3–Abnormalities of the hair, nails, and teeth
4–Occasional tapetoretinal degeneration

Horner's Syndrome
syn: Bernard-Horner syndrome
    Cervical sympathetic paralysis syndrome
1–Enophthalmos
2–Ptosis of upper eyelid
3–Miosis
4–Absence of sweating on the ipsilateral side of face and neck
5–Increased secretion of tears
6–Facial hemiatrophy

Howel-Evans Syndrome
1–Carcinoma of the esophagus
2–Keratosis palmaris and plantaris

Hunterian Glossitis Syndrome
1–Atrophic glossitis
2–Achylia gastrica
3–Primary macrocytic anemia

Hunter's Syndrome
1–Differs from Hurler's syndrome in milder course and no clouding of cornea
2–Excessive chondroitin sulfate and heparitin sulfate in urine
3–X-linked recessive trait

Hunt's Syndrome

syn: Ramsay-Hunt syndrome
1–Herpes zoster oticus
2–Facial palsy

Huriez's Syndrome

1–Sclerodermalike changes of the fingers
2–Atrophy of the backs of the hands
3–Palmar keratoderma
4–Squamous epitheliomas may develop in adolescence

Hurler-Pfaundler Syndrome

See Hurler's syndrome

Hurler's Syndrome

syn: Gargoylism
      Hurler-Pfaundler syndrome
1–Dwarfism with bizarre skeletal deformities
2–Hepatosplenomegaly
3–Clouding of cornea
4–Mental retardation
5–Deafness
6–Various cutaneous manifestations
    a. Specific papular and nodular lesions
    b. Thickening of skin of hands
    c. Hypertrichosis
7–Excessive chondroitin sulfate and heparitin
  sulfate in urine
8–Autosomal recessive trait

Hutchinson-Gilford Syndrome

syn: Premature senility syndrome
      Progeria syndrome
1–Infantilism with dwarfism
2–Alopecia: head, eyebrows, eyelashes
3–Premature aging

Hutchinson's Syndrome

syn: Hutchinson's triad
1–Interstitial keratitis
2–Eighth nerve deafness
3–Characteristic incisors and molars

Hutchinson's Triad

See Hutchinson's syndrome

Hydantoin Syndrome

syn: Pseudolymphoma syndrome
1–Morbilliform, scarlatiniform, urticarial or
    exfoliative eruptions
2–Fever, malaise, and arthralgia
3–Lymphadenopathy, particularly cervical nodes
4–Splenic or hepatic enlargement
5–Eosinophilia

Hydralazine Syndrome

1–Simulates systemic lupus erythematosus

Hypertrophied Frenuli Syndrome

See Oral-facial-digital syndrome

Hypoplastic Fingernail-Toenail Syndrome

1–Moderate to severe mental retardation
2–Unusually small nails
3–Various congenital defects
4–Partial trisomy

Idiopathic Familial Hyperlipemia Syndrome

See Bürger-Grütz syndrome

Incontinentia Pigmenti Syndrome
See Bloch-Sulzberger syndrome

Infantile Acrodermatitis Papulosa Syndrome
See Gianotti-Crosti syndrome

Intestinal Lipodystrophy Syndrome
See Whipple's syndrome

Iodide Fever Syndrome
1–Skin eruption
2–Fever
3–Coryza
4–Conjunctivitis
5–Lymphadenopathy

Islet-Cell Carcinoma of the Pancreas Syndrome
1–Transitory migratory annular erythema with
   superficial necrosis of the skin
2–Smooth red tongue
3–Mild diabetes
4–Normochromic anemia
5–Rapid weight loss

Jacob's Syndrome
See Oculo-oro-genital syndrome

Jacquet's Syndrome
1–Hypotrichosis of scalp
2–Congenital absence of nails
3–Dental anomalies

Jadassohn-Lewandowsky Syndrome
See Pachyonychia congenita syndrome

Jaffe's Syndrome
1–Mature angiomas of the skin
2–Similar vascular malformations in the abdominal viscera

Job's Syndrome
1–Recurrent cold staphylococcal abscesses

Joliffe's Syndrome
1–Nicotinic acid deficiency

Jung-Vogel Syndrome
1–Ichthyosis vulgaris
2–Diffuse palmoplantar keratosis
3–Anhidrosis
4–Corneal dystrophy

Kasabach-Merritt Syndrome
See Hemangioma-thrombocytopenia syndrome

Kast-Maffucci Syndrome
See Maffucci's syndrome

Kast's Syndrome
See Maffucci's syndrome

Keratoma Hereditaria Mutilans
See Vohwinkel's syndrome

Kernicterus Syndrome
See Crigler-Najjar syndrome

Kettle Syndrome
1–Lymphedema of lower extremity
2–Lymphangiosarcoma

Kinky Hair Syndrome
1–Peculiar kinky hair
2–Mental and motor retardation
3–Clonic seizures
4–Failure to thrive
5–Males only

Klauder's Syndrome
See Stevens-Johnson syndrome

Klippel-Feil Syndrome
1–Shortness of neck
2–Limitation of head movements
3–Growth of hair low down on neck

Klippel-Trenaunay-Weber Syndrome
1–Congenital angiomatosis of an extremity
2–Varicose veins of the extremity dating from
   infancy or birth
3–Developmental hypertrophy of underlying bone and
   soft structures

Kloepfer's Syndrome

1–Complete blindness beginning at about two months of age
2–Blistering after exposure to sun
3–Arrest of growth at age of 5-6 years
4–Progressive mental retardation

Kumer-Loos Syndrome

See Pachyonychia congenita syndrome

Kwashiorkor Syndrome

1–Edema
2–Depigmentation of hair and skin
3–Failure of growth
4–Various dermatoses

Laband's Syndrome

1–Hereditary gingival fibromatosis
2–Lysis of distal phalanges
3–Nail dysplasia
4–Possibly hepatosplenomegaly

Lassueur–Graham Little Syndrome

See Graham Little syndrome

Lawford's Syndrome

1–Facial port-wine stain
2–Chronic simple glaucoma
3–May be unilateral or bilateral

Lawrence-Seip Syndrome

See Lipoatrophic diabetes syndrome

Lazy-Leukocyte Syndrome
1–Recurrent stomatitis
2–Otitis
3–Gingivitis
4–Lowgrade fever
5–Severe peripheral neutropenia

Leopard Syndrome
See Multiple lentigines syndrome

Leprechaunism
See Donohue's syndrome

Leriche Syndrome
1–Necrosis in extremities secondary to occlusion of the femoral artery within the pelvis

Leschke's Syndrome
1–General weakness
2–Numerous brownish macules
3–Hyperglycemia

Lesch-Nyhan Syndrome
1–Hyperuricemia
2–Self-mutilation
3–Severe mental retardation
4–Choreoathetosis
5–Spastic cerebral palsy

Letterer-Siwe Syndrome
1–Cutaneous changes
- a. Hemorrhagic manifestations
- b. Maculopapular or papular lesions
- c. Typical seborrheic dermatitis
- d. Moist erosions and ulcers

2–Hepatosplenomegaly
3–Generalized lymphadenopathy
4–Eosinophilic granuloma of the bone

Libman-Sacks Syndrome
1–Systemic lupus erythematosus
2–Verrucous endocarditis

Lindau Disease
See von Hippel-Lindau syndrome

Lipoatrophic Diabetes Syndrome
syn: Berardinelli's syndrome
Lawrence-Seip syndrome

1–Generalized and marked wasting of subcutaneous fat
2–Nonketotic insulin-resistant diabetes
3–"Acromegaloid" overgrowth
4–Hepatomegaly, sometimes splenomegaly
5–Generalized muscular hypertrophy
6–Hypertrichosis
7–Hyperpigmentation
8–Hypertension
9–Corneal opacities
10–Elevated metabolic rate
11–Hyperlipemia

Lipomelanotic Reticulosis Syndrome
See Pautrier-Woringer syndrome

Lobstein's Syndrome
1–Fragility of bones and laxity of ligaments
2–Blue sclerae and often precocious arcus senilis
3–Otosclerosis
4–Defects in dental enamel
5–Unusual fineness of hair

Löfgren's Syndrome
1–Erythema nodosum
2–Bilateral hilar lymphadenopathy
3–Acute iritis
4–Tuberculin anergy or hypoergy

Lorain-Levi Syndrome
syn: Pituitary nanism syndrome
1–Dwarfism
2–Infantilism
3–Absence of pubic and axillary hair
4–Premature aging of skin

Louis Bar Syndrome
See Ataxia-telangiectasia syndrome

Lubarsch-Pick Syndrome
1–Atypical amyloidosis with macroglossia

Lyell's Syndrome
See Scalded skin syndrome

Maffucci's Syndrome
syn: Bean-Maffucci syndrome
Dyschondroplasia with hemagiomas syndrome
Kast-Maffucci syndrome
Kast's syndrome
1–Multiple hemangiomas of the skin, mucosae, and internal organs
2–Bone lesions
3–Dyschondroplasia
4–Phleboliths

Malignant Atrophic Papulosis
See Degos' syndrome

Malignant Down Syndrome
1–Acquired hypertrichosis lanuginosa
2–Internal carcinoma

Malignant Granulomatous Syndromes of Childhood
1–Eczematoid dermatitis of central part of face
2–Chronic suppurative lymphadenitis
3–Hepatosplenomegaly
4–Infiltration of pulmonary tissue

Marchesani's Syndrome
1–Short, stocky, well developed stature
2–Thick skin and hair
3–Hands spadelike with short stubby fingers
4–Various ocular abnormalities

Marfanoid Hypermobility Syndrome
1–Marfanoid habitus
2–Generalized hypermobility of the joints
3–Marked hyperextensibility of the skin

Marfan's Syndrome

syn: Arachnodactyly
1–Skeletal abnormalities, notably arachnodactyly
2–Ocular lesions
3–Cardiovascular disease
4–Striae atrophicae
5–Deficiency of subcutaneous fat

Margolis Syndrome

1–Sex-linked deaf mutism
2–Piebaldness
3–X-linked recessive inheritance

Marinesco-Sjögren Syndrome

1–Cerebellar ataxia
2–Mental and physical retardation
3–Cataract
4–Scalp hair fine, sparse, short and deficient in pigment
5–Thin, brittle fingernails

Maroteaux-Lamy Syndrome

1–Differs from Hurler's syndrome in severe osseous changes and normal intellect
2–Excessive amounts of chondroitin B in the urine
3–Autosomal recessive

Marshall-White Syndrome

1–Localized areas of ischemia of the palms
2–Periodic attacks of insomnia
3–Sinus arrhythmia

Mastocytosis Syndrome

1–Urticaria pigmentosa
2–Hepatosplenomegaly
3–Generalized lymphadenopathy
4–Osteolytic or sclerotic changes in the bones
5–Symptoms resembling those of carcinoid syndrome

McCarthy-Shklar Syndrome

1–Pyostomatitis vegetans
2–Ulcerative colitis

McKusick's Syndrome

syn: Cartilage-hair hypoplasia
1–Dwarfism
2–Fine hair
3–Immunological incompetence

Melanophoric Nevus Syndrome

See Naegeli's syndrome

Melkersson-Rosenthal Syndrome

1–Recurring facial paralysis or paresis
2–Edema and granuloma formation of lips
3–Scrotal tongue

Mendes Da Costa's Syndrome (1)

syn: Erythrokeratodermia variabilis
1–Variable bizarre geographic hyperkeratotic plaques
2–Independent areas of erythroderma

Mendes Da Costa's Syndrome (2)

1–Tense bullae on the trunk and limbs
2–Reticulate pigmentation with macular atrophy
3–Alopecia
4–Mental and physical retardation

Menkes' Syndrome

1–Small stature
2–Severe mental retardation
3–Epilepsy
4–Twisted and fractured stubby white hair
5–Inconstant aminoaciduria

Metastasizing Lipase-Forming Pancreatic Adenoma Syndrome

1–Polyarthritis
2–Nonsuppurating panniculitis
3–Eosinophilia

Meyer-Schwickerath-Grüterich-Weyers Syndrome

See Dysplasia oculodentodigitalis syndrome

Mikulicz's Syndrome

1–Bilateral painless enlargement of salivary and lacrimal glands
2–Xerostomia
3–Decrease in or absence of lacrimation

Milian's Syndrome

1–Fever and systemic manifestations
2–Ninth day erythema after the first injection of an arsphenamine

Milroy's Disease
See Nonne-Milroy-Meige syndrome

Mondor's Syndrome
1–Phlebitis of superficial veins of the pectoral region

Mongolism
See Down's syndrome

Monilethrix Syndrome
1–Spindle hair formation
2–Keratosis pilaris
3–Koilonychia

Montgomery's Syndrome
1–Xanthoma disseminatum

Morgagni's Syndrome
1–Almost entirely in women
2–Symmetrical benign thickening of the inner table of the frontal bone of the skull
3–Obesity
4–Hirsutism and other signs of virilism
5–Neuropsychiatric symptoms
6–Progressive visual failure

Morquio's Syndrome
1–Differs from Hurler's syndrome by severe bone changes of distinctive types and aortic regurgitation
2–Intellect may be normal or impaired
3–Keratosulfaturia
4–Autosomal recessive trait

Morvan's Syndrome

1–Recurrent painless whitlows
2–Syringomyelia or occasionally leprosy

Moschcowitz's Syndrome

syn: Thrombotic thrombocytopenic purpura
1–Thrombocytopenia (purpura)
2–Hemolytic anemia (jaundice, pallor)
3–Disturbance of the central nervous system

Moynahan's Syndrome

1–Multiple symmetrical mottling with moles
2–Genital hypoplasia
3–Stunted growth
4–Psychic infantilism despite normal intellect
5–Congenital mitral stenosis

Mucha-Habermann Syndrome

syn: Pityriasis lichenoides et varioliformis acuta
syndrome
1–Fever, malaise, and lymphadenopathy
2–Macules, vesicles, and papulonecrotic lesions which
leave varioliform scars

Muckle-Wells Syndrome

1–Recurrent urticaria
2–Deafness
3–Nephritis
4–Amyloidosis

Mucocutaneous Ocular Syndrome

See Stevens-Johnson syndrome

Mucosal Respiratory Syndrome

1–Influenzalike symptoms or pneumonia
2–Manifestations of Stevens-Johnson syndrome

Multiple Lentigines Syndrome

syn: Cardiocutaneous syndrome
     Leopard syndrome
1–Multiple lentigines
2–Cardiac defects
3–Ocular hypertelorism
4–Abnormalities of genitalia
5–Retardation of growth
6–Deafness

Myotonia Dystrophia Syndrome

syn: Steinert's disease
1–Tonic spasm of muscle
2–Atrophy of skin, panniculus, and musculature
3–Hypogonadism
4–Hypotrichosis
5–Cataracts
6–Premature aging

Naegeli's Syndrome

syn: Franceschetti-Jadassohn syndrome
     Melanophoric nevus syndrome
1–Reticular pigmentation of skin
2–Yellowish spots on enamel of teeth
3–Hypohidrosis
4–Keratosis palmaris et plantaris
5–Keratosis pilaris

Nail-patella-elbow Syndrome

syn: Congenital iliac horns syndrome
Fong's syndrome
Hereditary onycho-osteodysplasia syndrome
1–Onychatrophy
2–Absent or rudimentary patellae
3–Congenital dislocation of head of radius
4–Iliac horns

Neonatal Cold Injury Syndrome

1–Feeding difficulty
2–Lethargy
3–Coldness to touch
4–Edema and, sometimes, sclerema
5–Immobility
6–Strikingly red hands, feet and cheeks
7–Rectal temperature under 33°C

Netherton's Syndrome

1–Congenital ichthyosiform erythroderma
2–"Bamboo" hairs
3–Atopy
4–Inconstant aminoaciduria

Nevoid Basal Cell Carcinoma Syndrome

syn: Gorlin's syndrome
Ward's syndrome
1–Multiple basal cell carcinomas
2–Dyskeratosis of the palms and soles with pitting
3–Multiple dental follicular cysts of the jaws
4–Skeletal changes: spina bifida, bifid ribs, etc.
5–Hypertelorism
6–Calcification of the falx cerebri

Nevus of Ota

See Oculocutaneous pigmentation syndrome

Nevus Sebaceus Syndrome

1–Linear nevus sebaceus
2–Epileptic seizures
3–Mental retardation

Niemann-Pick Syndrome

1–Malnutrition and retarded development
2–Hepatosplenomegaly
3–Occasional cutaneous xanthomas
4–Pigmentation of skin

Nonne-Milroy-Meige Syndrome

syn: Milroy's disease
1–Hereditary nonpitting edema of the legs

Oculocerebral-Hypopigmentation Syndrome

1–Ocular anomalies
2–Mental retardation
3–Spasticity
4–Athetoid movements
5–Cutaneous hypopigmentation resembling albinism
6–Growth retardation

Oculocutaneous Pigmentation Syndrome

syn: Nevus of Ota
1–Benign pigmentation of the skin of the face,
 ipsilateral eye and adnexa
2–Follows the distribution of the first and second
 divisions of the trigeminal nerve

Oculogenital Syndrome

See Oculo-oro-genital syndrome

Oculoglandular Syndrome of Parinaud

1–A granulomatous usually single lesion involving the conjunctiva of one eye
2–Swelling of a preauricular lymph node
3–Lethargy
4–Low grade fever

Oculo-oro-genital Syndrome

syn: Jacob's syndrome
      Oculogenital syndrome
1–Stomatitis with ulcers on buccal mucosa
2–Conjunctivitis and keratitis
3–Exfoliative dermatitis of scrotum
4–Diarrhea
5–Inadequate rice diet

"Oid-Oid" Disease

See Sulzberger-Garbe syndrome

Oral-facial-digital (OFD) Syndrome

syn: Gorlin-Psaume syndrome
      Hypertrophied frenuli syndrome
1–Abnormally developed frenuli
2–Pseudoclefts in upper lip, tongue, and palate
3–Mental retardation
4–Family trembling
5–Syndactyly
6–Alopecia
7–Granular appearance of the skin of the face

52

Osler's Disease
   See Rendu-Osler-Weber syndrome

Otopalatodigital Syndrome
   1–Deafness
   2–Cleft palate
   3–Digital anomalies
   4–Characteristic facies
   5–Generalized bone dysplasia

Pachydermoperiostosis
   See Touraine-Solente-Golé syndrome

Pachyonychia Congenita Syndrome
   syn: Jadassohn-Lewandowsky syndrome
        Kumer-Loos syndrome
   1–Thickening of nails
   2–Plantar and palmar bullae and keratoses
   3–Follicular papules on buttocks and extremities
   4–Leukoplakia oris
   5–Corneal dyskeratoses and cataracts

Painful Bruising Syndrome
   See Autoerythrocyte sensitization syndrome

Papillon-LeFèvre Syndrome
   1–Palmar and plantar hyperkeratosis
   2–Periodontosis with loss of teeth
   3–Calcification of the dura

Parkinson's Syndrome
1–Muscular rigidity
2–Immobile facies
3–Tremor
4–Abolition of associated and automatic movements
5–Salivation
6–Seborrheic dermatitis

Parotitis-herpangina-Coxsackie Virus Syndrome
1–Inflammation of parotid glands
2–Vesicular and ulcerative lesions in the faucial area
3–Presence of Coxsackie virus

Parry-Romberg Syndrome
1–Progressive hemifacial atrophy
2–Contralateral Jacksonian epilepsy
3–Trigeminal neuralgia
4–Changes in the eyes and hair

Pasini's Syndrome
1–Dystrophic epidermolysis bullosa
2–Persistent firm ivory-white perifollicular
papules and plaques on the trunk

Paterson-Kelly Syndrome
See Plummer-Vinson syndrome

Pautrier-Woringer Syndrome
syn: Lipomelanotic reticulosis syndrome
1–Generalized superficial lymphadenopathy
2–Chronic nonspecific pruritic skin disorder

Pemphigus Erythematosus Syndrome
See Senear-Usher syndrome

"Perineal" Syndrome
1–Intense pruritus
2–Excessive sweating of the perineum

Perniotic Syndrome
1–Elderly men
2–Violaceous plaques on fingers, toes, ears and nose
3–Neutropenia
4–Monocytosis

Petges-Clégat Syndrome
syn: Poikilodermatomyositis syndrome
1–Poikiloderma
2–Dermatomyositis

Peutz-Jeghers Syndrome
syn: Peutz's syndrome
      Peutz-Touraine syndrome
1–Melanin pigmentation in and about body orifices and on digits
2–Generalized intestinal polyposis

Peutz's Syndrome
See Peutz-Jeghers syndrome

Peutz-Touraine Syndrome
See Peutz-Jeghers syndrome

PHC Syndrome
syn: Böök's syndrome
1–Premolar aplasia
2–Hyperhidrosis
3–Canities prematura

Pierre Robin Syndrome
1–Micrognathia
2–Microglossia
3–Glossoptosis
4–Cleft palate
5–Fine, light-colored hair

Pincer Nail Syndrome
1–Excessive transverse curvature of the nail plate
2–Severe pain

Pituitary Nanism Syndrome
See Lorain-Levi syndrome

Pityriasis Lichenoides et Varioliformis Acuta Syndrome
See Mucha-Habermann syndrome

Plummer-Vinson Syndrome
syn: Paterson-Kelly syndrome
1–Atrophy of the mucosa of mouth, tongue, pharynx, and esophagus
2–Dysphagia
3–Thinning of lips and angular cheilitis
4–Koilonychia
5–Microcytic hypochromic anemia
6–Middle-aged women

Poikiloderma Congenitale Syndrome
See Rothmund-Thomson syndrome

Poikilodermatomyositis Syndrome
See Petges-Clégat syndrome

Polydysplasia Syndrome

1–Progressive soft fatty subdermal masses
2–Pseudopapillomatosis around the orifices
3–Malformation of the distal extremities, especially congenital absence of the digits
4–Localized cutaneous aplasia
5–Other cutaneous anomalies

"Polyfibromatosis" Syndrome

1–Palmar fibromatosis
2–Knuckle pads
3–Plantar fibromatosis
4–Keloidal scarrings
5–Periarthritis of the shoulder
6–Plastic induration of the penis

Postphlebitic Syndrome

1–Thrombosis in the deep veins of the pelvis, thigh or leg
2–Edema
3–Development of collateral veins
4–Pigmentation
5–Induration, especially above internal malleolus
6–Characteristic dermatitis
7–Ulcer

Post-Traumatic Nevus Flammeus

See Fegeler's syndrome

Premature Senility Syndrome

See Hutchinson-Gilford syndrome

Pretibial Fever Syndrome
1–Erythematous rash in pretibial area
2–Mild respiratory symptoms
3–Febrile illness of five days' duration

Pringle's Syndrome
syn: Bourneville's syndrome
      Epiloia
1–Adenoma sebaceum
2–Epilepsy
3–Mental deficiency

Procainamide-Lupus Syndrome
1–Symptoms of systemic lupus erythematosus induced by procainamide

Profichet's Syndrome
See CRST syndrome

Progeria of the Adult Syndrome
See Werner's syndrome

Progeria Syndrome
See Hutchinson-Gilford syndrome

Pseudohypoparathyroidism
See Seabright-Bantam syndrome

Pseudolymphoma Syndrome
See Hydantoin syndrome

Pseudopseudohypoparathyroidism
See Seabright-Bantam syndrome

Psychogenic Purpura
See Autoerythrocyte sensitization syndrome

Purple People Syndrome
See Chlorpromazine syndrome

Purpura Hyperglobulinemica Syndrome
1–Recurrent dependent purpura
2–Hyperglobulinemia
3–Presence of rheumatoid factor

Ramsay-Hunt Syndrome
See Hunt's syndrome

Raynaud's Syndrome
1–Sequential blanching, cyanosis and redness of the hands and feet, especially the digits
2–Pain and stiffness of the joints
3–Sometimes superficial gangrene of digits

Refsum's Syndrome
1–Ichthyosis simplex
2–Chronic polyneuritis
3–Retinitis pigmentosa
4–Progressive nerve deafness
5–Cerebrospinal fluid shows albuminocytologic dissociation

Reiter's Syndrome
syn: Urethro-oculo-synovial syndrome
1–Polyarthritis
2–Conjunctivitis
3–Nonspecific urethritis
4–Cutaneous lesions resembling erythema multiforme or keratosis blennorrhagica

Relapsing Febrile Nodular Nonsuppurative Panniculitis Syndrome

See Weber-Christian syndrome

Rendu-Osler-Weber Syndrome

syn: Hereditary hemorrhagic telangiectasia
Osler's disease

1–Numerous telangiectases on skin and mucous membranes
2–Frequent or severe hemorrhage from the mucous membranes

Reye's Syndrome

1–Erythematous, occasionally papular or vesicular, eruption
2–Sudden vomiting
3–Fever
4–Convulsions
5–Coma

Richner-Hanhart Syndrome

1–Painful punctate palmoplantar keratoses
2–Prepatellar keratoses
3–Bradyphalangia
4–Herpetiform corneal dystrophy
5–Oligophrenia

Riley-Day Syndrome

syn: Familial autonomic dysfunction syndrome
Familial dysautonomia syndrome

1–Intermittent erythematous patches while eating or during excitement
2–Excessive perspiration
3–Drooling persisting beyond infancy
4–Failure to produce tears when crying

Riley-Smith Syndrome
1–Macrocephaly without hydrocephalus
2–Multiple subcutaneous and cutaneous hemangiomas
3–Pseudopapilledema

Romberg-Parry Syndrome
1–Facial hemiatrophy

Rosenthal-Kloepfer Syndrome
1–Corneal leukomata
2–Acromegaloid appearance
3–Cutis verticis gyrata

Rothmann-Makai Syndrome
1–Spontaneous circumscribed panniculitis

Rothmund-Thomson Syndrome
syn: Poikiloderma congenitale syndrome
1–Poikiloderma
2–Juvenile cataracts
3–Congenital bone defects
4–Disturbances of hair growth
5–Sensitivity to sunlight
6–Defective development of teeth and nails
7–Hypogonadism

Rowell-Beck-Anderson Syndrome
1–Discoid lupus erythematosus
2–Erythema-multiformelike lesions
3–Immunological abnormalities in the serum

Rubenstein-Taybi Syndrome
syn: Broad thumb and great toe syndrome
1–Broad thumb and great toes
2–Facial abnormalities
3–Psychomotor retardation
4–Highly arched palate

Rud's Syndrome
1–Ichthyosis simplex
2–Mental deficiency
3–Epilepsy
4–Infantilism

Ruiter-Pompen Syndrome
See Fabry-Anderson syndrome

Ruiter-Pompen-Wyers Syndrome
See Fabry-Anderson syndrome

Sanfilippo Syndrome
1–Differs from Hurler's syndrome in that somatic effects are mild, the CNS manifestations severe
2–Only heparitin sulfate is excreted in the urine in excess
3–Autosomal recessive trait

Savill's Syndrome
syn: Epidemic exfoliative dermatitis syndrome
1–Dry or moist exfoliative dermatitis of face, scalp, and upper limbs
2–Appears as epidemics in institutions

Scalded Skin Syndrome

syn: Lyell's syndrome
      Toxic epidermal necrolysis syndrome
1–Premonitory symptoms such as vomiting, diarrhea, and sore throat
2–Initial widespread erythema and edema
3–Extensive loosening of the skin with or without bullae
4–Denudation with raw red oozing surfaces sometimes involving practically the entire body
5–Extreme toxicity, frequently fatal

Scalenus Anticus Syndrome

syn: Cervical rib syndrome
1–Unilateral or bilateral cervical ribs
2–Pain, hyperesthesia, anesthesia, and paresthesia
3–Weakness and atrophy of muscles of the hands
4–Edema, coldness, pallor, and cyanosis of the hands
5–Diminution in pulse volume
6–At times, trophic ulcerations and gangrene

Schäfer-Siemens Syndrome

1–Hereditary palmo-plantar hyperkeratosis
2–Congenital cataract

Schaumann's Syndrome

1–Boeck's sarcoid
2–Hilus adenitis
3–Iridocyclitis
4–Osteitis multiplex cystoides

Scheie's Syndrome

1–Differs from Hurler's syndrome in stiff joints and aortic regurgitation
2–Intellect may be normal or impaired
3–Excessive amount of chondroitin B in the urine
4–Autosomal recessive

Schönlein-Henoch Syndrome
1–Nontraumatic hemorrhage in skin, subcutaneous tissue, and joints
2–Gastrointestinal pain and hemorrhage
3–Painful swelling of joints
4–Localized edema of backs of hands, face, or elsewhere
5–Hematuria and/or proteinuria

Scleredema Syndrome
1–Scleredema adultorum Buscke
2–Diabetes mellitus

Scleroderma-Calcinosis Syndrome
See CRST syndrome

Scleromyxedema
See Arndt-Gottron syndrome

Seabright-Bantam Syndrome
syn: Pseudohypoparathyroidism
Pseudopseudohypoparathyroidism
1–Lenticular calcification, cataracts, blue sclerae and strabismus
2–Decreased hearing and adherent ear lobes
3–Delayed dentition and/or dental aplasia
4–Subcutaneous calcifications and ossification
5–Various endocrinopathies
6–Multiple skeletal abnormalities
7–Oligophrenia

Senear-Usher Syndrome

syn: Pemphigus erythematosus syndrome
1–Lupus-erythematosuslike lesions on face
2–Crusted bullous lesions resembling impetigo contagiosa on chest and extremities
3–Changes related to seborrheic eczema
4–Positive Nikolsky sign

Sézary's Reticulosis Syndrome

See Sézary's syndrome

Sézary's Syndrome

syn: Sézary's reticulosis syndrome
1–Generalized exfoliative erythroderma
2–Intense pruritus
3–Pigmentation
4–Benign lymphadenopathy
5–Monocytosis
6–Alopecia
7–Splenomegaly

Shäfer's Syndrome

1–Pachyonychia congenita syndrome
2–Retardation of development with oligophrenia and hypogenitalism

Sheehan's Syndrome

1–Increasing lassitude
2–Loss of appetite
3–Wasting
4–Alopecia
5–Yellowish dry wrinkled skin

Shell Nail Syndrome
1–Shell-like deformity of the fingernails
2–Atrophy of the distal phalanges
3–Bronchiectasis

Shibi-Gacchyaki Syndrome
1–Undernutrition
2–Angular stomatitis
3–Cheilitis
4–Glossitis
5–Pellagralike skin lesions
6–Severe anogenital itching

Shoulder-Hand Syndrome
1–Painful shoulder disability
2–Homolateral vasomotor changes, with swelling of the hand
3–Later, dystrophic alterations of the hands and fingers

Sicca Syndrome
See Sjögren's syndrome

Sickle-cell Disease
syn: Dresbach's syndrome
    Herrick's syndrome
1–Chronic leg ulcers
2–Green sclerae
3–Pain in bones and joints
4–Weakness and dyspnea
5–Attacks of acute abdominal pain
6–Recurrent swelling of hands and feet in children

Siemens' Syndrome (1)

syn: Hereditary anhidrotic ectodermal dysplasia syndrome

1–Absence or paucity of sweat, sebaceous, and mucous glands
2–Hypotrichosis
3–Anodontia

Siemens' Syndrome (2)

See Bloch-Sulzberger syndrome

Silver's Syndrome

1–Shortness of stature
2–Congenital asymmetry
3–Premature sexual development
4–Café au lait spots occasionally

Simons' Syndrome

1–Progressive lipodystrophy

Sjögren-Larsson Syndrome

1–Congenital ichthyosiform erythroderma
2–Mental deficiency
3–Cerebral spastic diplegia
4–Frequently degenerative retinitis

Sjögren's Syndrome

syn: Gougerot-Mulock-Houwer syndrome
Gougerot-Sjögren syndrome
Sicca syndrome

1–Dryness of all the mucous membranes and skin
2–Rheumatoid arthritis
3–Anemia
4–Sometimes sclerodermalike changes, alopecia, or telangiectasia

Skin-eye Syndrome
See Chlorpromazine syndrome

Spannlang-Tappeiner Syndrome
1–Palmoplantar keratosis
2–Partial or total alopecia
3–Hyperhidrosis
4–Tongue shaped corneal opacities

Speransky-Richen-Siegmund Syndrome
1–Necrosis and sloughing in the oral cavity leading to perforation of the hard palate into the maxillary sinus, and detachment of the alveolar processes

Sphenopalatine Syndrome
1–Chronic and intermittent edema of the face
2–Lacrimation on the affected side
3–Unilateral rhinitis occasionally seen
4–Paroxysms of swelling alternating with erythema affecting side of bridge of the nose may occur

Spotted Leg Syndrome
1–Diabetes with retinopathy and/or neuropathy
2–Irregularly round or oval shallow or depressed atrophic brown patches on fronts and sides of legs

Steiner's Syndrome
See Curtius' syndrome

Steinert's Disease

See Myotonia dystrophia syndrome

Stein-Leventhal Syndrome

1–Bilateral polycystic ovaries
2–Amenorrhea or oligomenorrhea
3–Obesity
4–Sterility
5–Hirsutism

Stevens-Johnson Syndrome

syn: Ectodermosis erosiva pluriorificialis syndrome
Erythema multiforme exudativum major
syndrome
Fiessinger-Rendu syndrome
Klauder's syndrome
Mucocutaneous ocular syndrome

1–Fever and severe constitutional symptoms
2–Extensive stomatitis
3–Conjunctivitis, keratitis, uveitis, and even
panophthalmitis
4–Ulcerative lesions on mucosa of nose, penis, and
vagina, and about anus
5–Vesicobullous or petechial and hemorrhagic eruption on face, hands, and feet

Stewart's Syndrome

1–Oligophrenia
2–Ichthyosis
3–Retinitis pigmentosa
4–Arachnodactylia
5–Infantilism
6–Epilepsy

Stewart-Treves Syndrome
1–Edematous upper extremity after radical breast surgery
2–Lymphangiosarcoma

Stiff Skin Syndrome
1–Rock hard skin
2–Mild hirsutism
3–Joint stiffness

Still-Chauffard Syndrome
1–Arthritis of cervical spine
2–Anemia and leukopenia
3–Splenomegaly and lymphadenopathy
4–Cutaneous pigmentation, especially on cheeks

Stryker-Halbeisen Syndrome
1–Scaly and vesicular patches of erythroderma on face, neck, and upper chest
2–Intense pruritus
3–Macrocytic anemia

Sturge-Kalischer-Weber Syndrome
See Sturge-Weber syndrome

Sturge-Weber Syndrome
syn: Encephalotrigeminal angiomatosis syndrome
Sturge-Kalischer-Weber syndrome
1–Angiomas of the choroid and pia mater
2–Ipsilateral port-wine stain along the course of the superior and middle branches of the trigeminal nerve
3–Convulsions
4–Paralysis
5–Mental retardation
6–Visual disturbances

Sudeck's Syndrome
1–Acute pain
2–Atrophy of skin, subcutaneous tissue, and bone
3–These manifestations occur at site of minor injury

Sulzberger-Garbe Syndrome
syn: "Oid-oid" disease
1–Chronic exudative discoid and lichenoid dermatitis
2–Severe nocturnal pruritus
3–Chiefly middle-aged, neurotic, Jewish males

Superior Vena Cava Syndrome
1–Marked facial and eyelid edema
2–Band of dilated blood vessels around lower chest wall
3–Gynecomastia

Sweat Retention Syndrome
syn: Tropical anhidrotic asthenia syndrome
1–Anhidrosis
2–Miliaria
3–Attacks of pruritus
4–Severe systemic symptoms
5–Collapse

Sweet's Syndrome
syn: Acute febrile neutrophilic dermatosis
1–Fever
2–Variable degrees of headache, vomiting, abdominal pain and prostration
3–Raised painful plaques or nodules on the limbs, face, and neck
4–Sterile pustules
5–Neutrophilic polymorphonuclear leukocytosis

Swift's Syndrome
  See Feer's syndrome

Takahara's Syndrome
  syn: Acatalasemia
  1–Progressive gangrenous lesions involving the gingiva
    and alveolar bone
  2–Exfoliation of teeth

Tetralogy of Fallot Syndrome
  1–Group of congenital cardiac defects
  2–Cyanosis of lips and nail beds
  3–Clubbing of the fingers
  4–Gums are swollen and red
  5–May be telangiectases on cheeks

Teutschlaender Syndrome
  1–Calcinosis universalis

Thévenard's Syndrome
  syn: Familial mutilating ulcerous acropathy syndrome
      Familial ulceration of the extremities syndrome
  1–Trophic ulcers of soles
  2–Hypesthesia to pain and temperature on soles
  3–Osteodystrophies of the feet and spine

Thibierge-Weissenbach Syndrome
  See CRST syndrome

Thomas-Bureau Syndrome
  See Bureau-Barriere-Thomas syndrome

Thorson-Biörck Syndrome
See Carcinoid syndrome

Thost-Unna Syndrome
1–Diffuse palmoplantar keratoderma

Thrombotic Thrombocytopenic Purpura
See Moschcowitz's syndrome

Thyrohypophyseal Syndrome
1–Euthyroidism
2–Ocular manifestations suggestive of hyperthyroidism
3–Facial, temporal, and pretibial edema

Thyroid Acropachy Syndrome
1–Hyperthyroidism with exophthalmos
2–Pretibial myxedema
3–Clubbing and/or hypertrophic osteoarthropathy

Tietz Syndrome
1–Albinoidism
2–Deaf-mutism
3–Hypoplasia of the eyebrows

Tooth and Nail Syndrome
1–Absent or very small and spoon shaped nails
2–Missing teeth

Touraine-Solente-Golé Syndrome
syn: Pachydermoperiostosis
1–Cutis sulcata of scalp, forehead and face
2–Periosteal lesions and hypertrophy of long bones
3–Clubbing of fingers and toes

Toxic Epidermal Necrolysis Syndrome
See Scalded skin syndrome

Tricho-rhino-phalangeal Syndrome
1–Hypotrichosis
2–Pear shaped nose
3–Multiple cone-shaped epiphyses of the digits of the hands and feet

Trigeminal Trophic Syndrome
1–Ulceration following minor trauma to anesthetic skin within the trigeminal area

Triparanol Syndrome
1–Alopecia
2–Depigmentation of hair
3–Ichthyosis
4–Cataracts

Trisomy 18 Syndrome
1–Loose folds of skin with typical dermal patterns
2–Horizontal palmar creases and downy hair
3–Poor subcutaneous tissue
4–Multiple congenital anomalies

Trisomy 21 Syndrome
See Down's syndrome

Troissier's Syndrome
1–Bronzed cachexia
2–Diabetes mellitus

Tropical Anhidrotic Asthenia Syndrome
See Sweat retention syndrome

Turner's Syndrome
syn: Bonnevie-Ullrich syndrome
Ullrich-Turner syndrome
1–Webbed neck
2–Lymphangiectatic edema of hands and feet
3–Cutis laxa and hyperelastica
4–Mental and physical retardation
5–Variable multiple congenital abnormalities
6–Forty-five chromosomes (XO)

Ullrich-Turner Syndrome
See Turner's syndrome

Universal Alopecia Syndrome
1–Universal alopecia
2–Onychodystrophy
3–Pigmentation of skin
4–Gastrointestinal polyposis

Urethro-oculo-synovial Syndrome
See Reiter's syndrome

Uveomeningitis Syndrome
See Vogt-Koyanagi-Harada syndrome

Van Den Bosch's Syndrome
1–Acrokeratosis verruciformis
2–Hair and nail dystrophy
3–Anhidrosis
4–Dwarfism
5–Retinochoroidal dystrophy
6–Nystagmus
7–Myopia

Van der Hoeve's Syndrome
1–Blue sclerae
2–Brittle bones
3–Deafness
4–Frequently abnormalities of nails, hair, and dental enamel

van Lohuizen's Syndrome
1–Congenital generalized phlebectasia

Vogt-Koyanagi-Harada Syndrome
syn: Uveomeningitis syndrome
1–Bilateral uveitis with iritis and glaucoma
2–Retinochoroidal detachment
3–Signs of meningeal irritation with pleocytosis
4–Alopecia, vitiligo, and poliosis may be temporarily associated
5–Dysacousia
6–Deafness may occur

Vohwinkel's Syndrome
syn: Keratoma hereditaria mutilans
1–Diffuse palmoplantar keratoderma honeycombed by small depressions
2–Starfishlike keratoses on the dorsa of the hands and feet
3–Irregular linear keratoses of knees and elbows
4–Constricting fibrous bands on fingers and toes

Volavsek's Syndrome
1–Keratosis palmaris, involving chiefly the periarticular areas of the fingers
2–Syringomyelia
3–Nail dystrophy

von Hippel-Lindau Syndrome

syn: Angiomatosis retinae et cerebelli syndrome
Lindau disease

1–Angiomatosis of retinae and cerebellum
2–Tumors and cysts of various organs
3–Rarely, vascular nevi of face

Waardenburg-Klein Syndrome

See Waardenburg's syndrome

Waardenburg's Syndrome

syn: Waardenburg-Klein syndrome

1–Pigmentary disturbances including partial albinism, white forelock, and partial or complete heterochromia iridum
2–Congenital deafness
3–Fused thick eyebrows, broad nasal root, and laterally displaced inner canthi

Waldenström's Syndrome

1–Relapsing nonthrombocytopenic purpura
2–Xerostomia and xerophthalmia
3–Hepatosplenomegaly and lymphadenopathy
4–Mild anemia
5–High erythrocyte sedimentation rate
6–Marked increase in serum gamma globulin
7–Rarely, infiltrated cutaneous and mucosal nodules and plaques

Ward's Syndrome

See Nevoid basal cell carcinoma syndrome

Waterhouse-Friderichsen Syndrome
1–Cyanosis
2–Purpuric macules
3–Meningococcal septicemia

Watson Syndrome
1–Multiple café au lait spots
2–Pulmonary valvular stenosis
3–Dull intelligence

Weber-Christian Syndrome
syn: Relapsing febrile nodular nonsuppurative panniculitis syndrome
1–Recurrent attacks of malaise and fever
2–Localized inflammatory subcutaneous nodules
3–Subcutaneous atrophy at the sites of nodules

Weber-Cockayne Syndrome
1–Epidermolysis bullosa simplex limited to hands and
feet

Weech's Syndrome
See Christ-Siemens syndrome

Wegener's Granulomatosis Syndrome
See Wegener's syndrome

Wegener's Syndrome
syn: Wegener's granulomatosis syndrome
1–Severe sinopulmonary inflammation
2–Generalized necrotizing angiitis
3–Symmetrical papulonecrotic lesions of extremities
4–Widespread vesicular or urticarial lesions
5–Pyoderma gangrenosum
6–Terminal renal insufficiency

Werner's Syndrome
syn: Progeria of the adult syndrome
1–Premature graying and loss of hair
2–Atrophy of the skin and subcutaneous tissue
3–Precocious cataracts
4–Endocrine disturbances

Whipple's Syndrome
syn: Intestinal lipodystrophy syndrome
1–Arthritis
2–Abdominal symptoms
3–Diarrhea with evidence of steatorrhea
4–Cough
5–Loss of weight
6–Asthenia
7–Patchy brown pigmentation of the skin
8–Purpura

Wiedemann-Beckwith Syndrome
1–Fine short lightly pigmented sparse hair
2–Variable intelligence
3–Macrosomia
4–Macroglossia

Wildervanck's Syndrome
See Cervico-oculo-acoustic syndrome

Willan-Plumbe Syndrome
1–Psoriasis

Wilson's Syndrome
syn: Hepatolenticular degeneration syndrome
1–Kayser-Fleischer rings
2–Azure lunulae of nails
3–Behavior disorders frequent
4–Disturbance in copper metabolism

Wiskott-Aldrich Syndrome

syn: Aldrich's syndrome
1–Thrombocytopenic purpura
2–Chronic eczema
3–Recurrent purulent infections

Wissler's Syndrome

1–High intermittent fever
2–Irregularly recurring macular or maculopapular exanthemata
3–Polymorphonuclear leukocytosis, often eosinophilia
4–Raised erythrocyte sedimentation rate

Witkop-Sallmann Syndrome

See Hereditary benign intraepithelial dyskeratosis syndrome

Wright's Syndrome

See Albright's syndrome

Wyburn-Mason Syndrome

1–Arteriovenous aneurysm of the midbrain
2–Congenital anomalies of the retinal vessels of one side
3–Telangiectatic nevus in the skin in the region of the affected eye

XTE Syndrome

1–Xeroderma
2–Talipes
3–Enamel defect

"Yellow Nail" Syndrome

1–Slow growing discolored nails
2–Edema, usually of the ankles
3–Pleural effusion

Zinsser-Cole-Engman Syndrome
See Dyskeratosis congenita syndrome

Zinsser-Fanconi Syndrome
See Dyskeratosis congenita syndrome

Ziprkowski-Adam Syndrome
1–Recessive total albinism
2–Congenital deaf-mutism

Index

83

Hand(s), *(cont.)*
  edema, coldness, pallor and
    cyanosis of, 63
  injuries of, 15
  spadelike, 43
  swelling of, 29, 66
  thickening of skin on, 34
  vasomotor changes in, 66
Hay fever, 3
Head, limitation of movements, 38
Headache, 71
Head injury, history of, 23
Heart, defects of, 24, 26, 78
  congenital, 21, 49, 72
  disease, 13, 44
  enlargement, 22
  lesions of, 5
  pulmonary stenosis, 78
Hemangioma, 31, 43, 61
  bluish, bladderlike, 7
  intestinal, bleeding from, 7
  spinal cord, 14
Hematoma, palm, 1
Hematuria, 64
Hemiatrophy, facial, 33, 54, 61
Hemihypertrophy, of body, 16
  of face, 16
Hemiplegia, 9, 32
Hemorrhage, 27, 41, 64, 69
  gastrointestinal, 5, 7
  from mucous membranes, 60
  mucocutaneous, 25
Heparitin sulfate, in urine, 33, 34, 62
Hepatomegaly, 35, 41
Hepatosplenomegaly, 10, 12, 16, 25, 34, 39, 41, 43, 45, 51, 77
Herniation of adipose tissue, 24
Herpes zoster, ophthalmicus, 32
  oticus, 34
Herpetiform plaques, 9
Hilus adenitis, 63
Hirsutism, 8, 16, 18, 47, 69, 70
  facial, in women, 1
Hydrocephalus, 61
Hyperelasticity of skin, 20
Hyperesthesia, 23, 63
Hyperextensibility of joints, 20
Hyperglobulinemia, 59
Hyperglycemia, 40

Hyperhidrosis, 9, 12, 16, 27, 29, 55, 60, 68
  of cheeks while eating, 5
  palmar and plantar, 24
  of perineum, 55
  See also Sweating
Hyperkeratosis, geographic plaques, 45
  palmar and plantar, 13, 53
Hyperlipemia, 41
Hyperpigmentation, 16, 41
  See also Pigmentation
Hypertelorism, 49, 50
Hypertension, 1, 16, 22, 31, 41
Hyperthyroidism, 73
  with exophthalmos, 73
Hypertrichosis, 19, 34, 41, 43
Hypertrophy of long bones, 73
Hyperuricemia, 40
Hypervitaminosis-A, 10
Hypesthesia, 72
Hypoergy, tuberculin, 42
Hypogenitalism, 65
Hypogonadism, 49, 61
Hypohidrosis, 6, 31, 49
Hypopigmentation, 51
Hypoplasia of eyebrows, 73
Hypopyon, 6
Hypothermia, 50
  attacks of, 32
Hypotrichosis, 13, 20, 27, 29, 49, 67, 74
  of eyebrows, 20, 24, 26
  of eyelashes, 20, 24
  of scalp, 36

Ichthyosiform erythroderma, congenital, 50, 67
Ichthyosis, 14, 17, 69, 74
  simplex, 37, 59, 62
Icterus, chronic idiopathic, 19
  retention, 15
Iliac horns, 50
Immobility, 50
Immunological abnormalities, 61
Immunological incompetence, 45
Impetigo contagiosa, 65
Induration, above internal malleolus, 57
Infantilism, 34, 42, 62, 69
  psychic, 48
Infections, recurrent purulent, 80

sinopulmonary, 4
Influenza, 49
Insomnia, 44
Intestinal polyposis, 55
Iridocyclitis, 6, 63
Iris, heterochromia of, 77
Iritis, 42, 76
Itching, 9
  See also Pruritus

Jaundice, 48
Jewish males, middle-aged neurotic, 71
Joints, enlargement of, 5
  hyperextensibility of, 20
  hypermobility of, 43
  painful, swelling of, 64
  stiff, contracted, 14
  stiffness of, 70

Kayser-Fleischer rings, 79
Keloids, 57
Keratitis, 52, 69
  dendritic, 30
  interstitial, 35
Keratoderma climactericum, 31
Keratosis(es), of arms and legs, 28
  of dorsa of hands and feet, 28, 76
  of knees and elbows, 76
  palmar, 34, 76
  palmar and plantar, 2, 6, 9, 10, 13, 16, 24, 28, 29, 30, 33, 37, 49, 53, 60, 63, 68, 73, 76
  prepatellar, 60
Keratosis blennorrhagica, 59
Keratosis pilaris, 47, 49
Keratosulfaturia, 47
Kidney, disease of, 17, 29
Knuckle pads, 5, 57
Koilonychia, 47, 56, 73

Labia majora, hypoplasia of, 27
Labial glands, hyperplastic, 4
Lacrimal glands, enlargement of, 31, 46
Lacrimation, absence of, 46
  decrease in, 12, 46
  and facial palsy, 15
  paroxysmal, 15
  unilateral, 68
Lassitude, 65
Leg(s), edema of, 22

induration of, 57
  ulcers of, 22, 24, 57
Lens, deposits in, 12
  star shaped opacities, 12
Lentigines, multiple, 49
Leprosy, 48
Lethargy, 50, 52
Leukocytes, inclusions in, 12
Leukocytosis, eosinophilic, 80
  neutrophilic, 71, 80
Leukoma, corneal, 61
Leukonychia, total, 5
Leukopenia, 24, 70
Leukoplakia oris, 19, 53
Lichen myxedematosus, 4
Lichen planus, 28
Ligaments, laxity of, 42
Light sensitivity, 7, 30, 39, 61
Lip(s), bullous lesions on, 7
  double, acquired, 4
  edema of, 45
  granuloma formation of, 45
  hyperplasia of glands of, 4
  thinning of, 56
Lipemia retinalis, 10
Lipodystrophy, 67
Lipoma(s), 18, 30, 57
Liver, cirrhosis of, 16, 30, 31
  discoloration of, 19
  enlargement of, 35
Lung(s), infiltration of, 43
Lunulae, azure, of nails, 79
Lupus erythematosus, 7, 14, 35, 41, 58, 61, 65
Lymphadenitis, chronic suppurative, 43
Lymphadenopathy, 11, 12, 21, 24, 26, 35, 36, 41, 45, 48, 52, 54, 65, 70, 77
  hilar, 42, 63
Lymphangiectasis, 75
Lymphangiosarcoma, 38, 70

Macrocephaly, 61
Macroglossia, 42, 79
Macrosomia, 79
Macular atrophy, 46
Malaise, 26, 35, 48, 78
Malignancy, of vascular endothelium, 3
Malignant disease, 25
Malnutrition, 27, 51

89

91